"[...]
p[...]
It [...]"

Exeter, New Hampshire

"A great asthma resource."

Tim Rumsey, M.D., Family Practitioner
Saint Paul, Minnesota

" *One Minute Asthma* helps me explain that triggers are long-lasting and add up."

Gary Brecher, M.D., Pediatrician
Rockville, Maryland

"New patients who have read a few pages of *One Minute Asthma* in the waiting room are easier to talk to than those who haven't."

Jane Purser, M.D., Allergist
Tulsa, Oklahoma

"I use *One Minute Asthma* to convince parents that inhaled steroids can safely prevent most of their child's attacks."

G. Bradley Gascoigne III, M.D., Pediatrician
Cleveland, Ohio

"I use *One Minute Asthma* as an outline for my workshops with school staff and parents, and I give each a copy to take home."

Frances Belmonte-Mann, RN, MA, School Nurse Administrator
Chicago, Illinois

One Minute
ASTHMA

What You Need to Know

Thomas F. Plaut, M.D.

Pedipress, Inc.
Amherst, Massachusetts

NOTICE

The information in this book is general and may not apply to your specific situation.

DO NOT CHANGE YOUR MEDICINE ROUTINE WITHOUT CONSULTING YOUR DOCTOR.

In print

English edition	*1,830,000 copies*
Spanish edition	*170,000 copies*

Edited by Suzanne Plaut and Stacey Velez
Illustrated by Carla Brennan

Library of Congress Cataloging-in-Publication Data

Plaut, Thomas F., 1933-
  One minute asthma : what you need to know /
Thomas F. Plaut.-- 7th ed.
      p. cm.
  ISBN 0-914625-28-4 (paperback)
  1. Asthma--Popular works. I. Title.
  RC591.P53 2005
  616.2'38--dc22

                                    2005045917

Contents

Introduction

For Doctors

Busy doctors told me they wanted to teach their patients about asthma in their office and the ER. But they could find no easy-to-read book on asthma. I wrote *One Minute Asthma* to solve this problem. Each page presents a single concept or set of facts to the patient or parent. Patients can read a few pages in your waiting room, exam room or at home. After reading, they will ask better questions and have a more focused visit.

For Parents, Teens and Adults

The word "asthma" scares a lot of people. In the past, asthma was hard to treat. Today asthma treatment is very good. Most people with asthma should be able to do everything they want to do.

This book can help you to stay out of the ER and the hospital. First, learn the basics of asthma and the medicines used to treat it. Second, track your asthma using peak flow or asthma signs scores. After you do this, you and your doctor can work out a clear action plan for treating your asthma at home.

Thomas F. Plaut, M.D.
Amherst, Massachusetts
2005

You Can Control Asthma

You and your doctor should work out a good plan to control your asthma. Then you will be able to:
- Run as fast and as long as you want.
- Sleep through the night without a cough or wheeze.
- Attend school or work *every* day.
- Avoid urgent visits to the doctor.
- Stay out of the ER.

Your asthma is out of control if you have symptoms or use a rescue medicine (med) more than two days each week. You and your doctor need to learn more about your asthma. Then you can work out a better plan.

Danger Signs of Asthma

Go to the ER or call 911 right away if you notice any one of these signs:
- You hunch over when you breathe.
- Your lips or the tips of your fingers are blue.
- You have trouble walking or talking.
- You are sucking in the skin between your ribs.
- You are breathing very slowly.

How to Find a Good Asthma Doctor

If your asthma is under control, you will probably never have a severe asthma problem.

To find a good asthma doctor, look for someone who:

- Expects you to achieve excellent control of your asthma.
- Works with you as a partner to control your asthma.
- Teaches you how to reduce asthma triggers at home, school and work.
- Measures your peak flow or lung function each time you visit.
- Shows you how to take your inhaled meds and checks your technique. (The office staff may do this.)
- Writes down the dose, timing and technique for giving or taking meds.

If your regular doctor does not do these things, ask to see an asthma specialist.

Signs of Asthma Trouble

There are four main signs of asthma:

Cough. Worse at night, after exercise, in a smoky room or in cold air.

Wheeze. A whistling noise heard when breathing out.

Breathing much faster or slower than usual. Count your breathing rate for 30 seconds. Compare this to your rate when you are well.

Sucking in the chest skin. You can see this between the ribs and at the front of the neck.

If you notice any one of these signs, avoid triggers and start or increase your asthma meds.

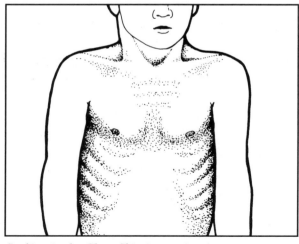

Sucking in the Chest Skin (retractions)

What is Asthma?

Asthma is a long-standing (chronic) disease. When you have asthma, your airways are over-sensitive and inflamed.

Asthma is often called wheezy bronchitis, asthmatic bronchitis, bronchial asthma or reactive airway disease (RAD). Doctors may call asthma acute bronchitis or pneumonia. If you have been told that you have bronchitis or pneumonia more than once in a year, you probably have asthma.

The words "asthma problem," "asthma episode," "asthma attack" and "asthma flare" all mean the same thing.

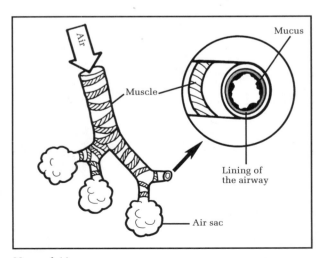

Normal Airway

What Happens in the Airways?

The tubes that carry air into the lungs are called "airways" or "bronchioles." They are more sensitive in people with asthma. They react to asthma triggers such as colds, cigarette smoke and exercise faster and more strongly than normal airways. During an asthma problem:

- The airway lining becomes inflamed, swells and makes more mucus. This narrows the airways and reduces the air flow.
- The muscles around the airways tighten. This lowers air flow more.

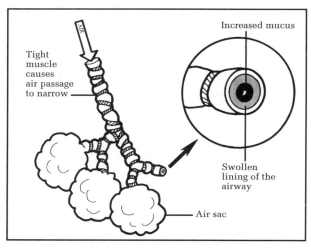

Airway During Episode

Asthma Triggers

A trigger is any object, act or event that makes the airways more sensitive or inflamed, or that causes asthma symptoms. The effects of triggers may last many days and they may add up. This means that a second trigger will cause worse symptoms if your airways are still inflamed. Here are some common triggers:

- Exercise
- Viral infections (cold, bronchitis, pneumonia)
- Pollution (such as cigarette smoke, smoke from a wood stove, perfume or dust)
- Allergens (such as cats, dogs, mites, cockroaches, grass, mold and pollen)
- Cold air
- Coughing, yelling and laughing
- Some medicines and chemicals.

Exercise is one trigger you should not avoid.

Triggers have Effects that are Long-lasting and Add Up

The graph below shows three areas. People with normal airways are in area A. People with asthma always have airways that over-react. They are in area B. Being near a cat causes the airways to be more sensitive. As a result, symptoms appear. This occurs in area C. In this example, symptoms are gone within ten days. But the airways are still over-sensitive. This makes a person more likely to react to other triggers. If a person then gets a head cold, asthma symptoms will show up again and will last even longer.

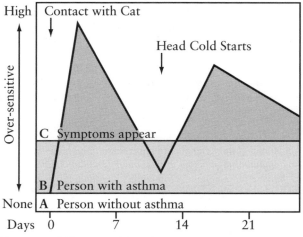

Triggers and Over-sensitive airways

Triggers in the Home

To help control asthma, do as many of these things as you can:

- Do not let people smoke in your house or car.
- If you are allergic to your pet, find a new home for it, keep it outside or wash it with tap water every week.
- Keep the humidity in your house between 25 and 50 percent (to reduce growth of mold).
- Remove wall-to-wall carpets.
- Use double thickness vacuum cleaner bags.
- Use a HEPA air filter in the bedroom.
- Encase your mattress, box spring and pillows in anti-allergic covers (to keep dust mites out of them).
- Cover heating vents with an air filter.
- Use an air conditioner (to reduce allergens, pollutants and humidity).
- Use boric acid (not a spray) to kill roaches.
- Put stuffed animals in the freezer overnight (to kill dust mites).
- Use an exhaust fan in the bathroom (to reduce humidity).
- Use a hood over the stove (to vent cooking fumes).
- Vent the clothes dryer to the outside (to reduce humidity).

Exercise is one trigger you should not avoid.

Triggers in the School

If your child has asthma, work with other parents and adults at the school. Be sure that your school keeps dirt, dust, debris and odors from entering the building. Be sure the community supports the maintenance budget. Also make sure that all of the following are true:

- The heating, ventilating and air conditioning (HVAC) system has been cleaned and checked. It should work according to the manufacturer's specifications.
- The school uses hard-surface flooring that is easy to clean and maintain when they replace carpets or build a new school. (Wall-to-wall carpets let molds and mites breed. They also adsorb pollutants. Schools cannot clean these carpets well enough.)
- Low odor products are used in classes. All fumes are vented. (Often gasses are released in art class, metal or woodworking shop and science labs. Office machines, like copiers and printers, pollute the air near where they are placed.)
- School buses do not idle outside the school longer than allowed by city or state law (often 3-5 minutes). The buses' exhaust may be sucked up by air intake vents. Then your child breathes in the exhaust. Check your local laws.

- The pest control and cleaning materials used in the school and yard are low odor and low toxicity.
- New flooring and furnishings are made of low odor materials. Let them off-gas before students go near them.

For more information, contact the Healthy Schools Network (see Resource Section).

Exercise

Exercise is the most common asthma trigger. When your asthma is well controlled, you can play any sport and run as fast and as long as anyone else, except during an episode.

Your asthma plan is not good enough if exercise causes any of these symptoms:
- Cough,
- A tight chest,
- Wheeze.

If these symptoms happen within six minutes of starting hard exercise, your asthma is not controlled. You need a new treatment plan.

If your symptoms happen only after at least six minutes of hard exercise, you have exercise induced asthma. Pretreat with a rescue med, then warm up to prevent symptoms.

Sinus Trouble

The sinuses are air pockets in the bones of the face and the skull behind it. When they become inflamed, they can trigger an asthma problem. They can also prevent an asthma problem from clearing. Sinusitis may cause a headache, pain when you bend over, pain in the teeth or a colored discharge from the nose.

The sinuses produce mucus that drains into the nose. When inflamed, the sinuses produce more mucus. If this mucus cannot drain, the sinuses may become infected. To prevent this:

- Rinse your nose daily at the first sign of a cold. Use salt water (one half teaspoon of salt in eight ounces of warm water). Inhale one ounce (several sniffs) into each nostril from a cup or use a "neti-pot" or a bulb syringe.
- Take an inhaled nasal steroid or an antihistamine during your allergy season.

To reduce symptoms that you have:

- Rinse your nose two to three times a day. This will unclog the opening to the sinuses and help them drain.
- Use a decongestant.

If your sinusitis gets worse, see your doctor.

Allergic Rhinitis

An inflamed nose (rhinitis) may cause asthma symptoms to appear or make them last longer. The symptoms are sneezing, a runny nose or a blocked nose. If you have these symptoms often, get a skin or blood test to find out what causes them. Then find a way to expose yourself less to these triggers.

Treatment with an antihistamine or decongestant can reduce your symptoms. You can also inhale a nasal steroid or cromolyn into your nose every day. This often will reduce the number of times you have rhinitis.

Coughing and Asthma

Coughing is often the first sign that your asthma is not under control. People with asthma often cough in the following situations:

- At night,
- With exercise,
- In smoky areas,
- After laughing or crying and
- In cold air.

Use your asthma medicine to control your cough. It is not safe to take only a cough medicine without treating your asthma.

How Severe is Your Asthma?

To assess your **long term asthma status**, doctors check how often you had asthma symptoms when you were not taking any asthma meds.

If you had asthma symptoms or used a quick relief med 0 - 2 days a week (on average) you have **mild intermittent asthma**. You should reduce the triggers in your home, car and office. You will need to take meds only to relieve symptoms.

If you had symptoms like a slight cough, wheeze or tight chest more than two days a week, you have **persistent asthma**. You need to reduce triggers and take meds every day. There are three levels:

- If you have symptoms three to six days a week, you have *mild persistent asthma*. Usually you can avoid symptoms by taking an inhaled steroid every day.
- If you have symptoms every day, you have *moderate persistent asthma*. You may have to take two controller (control) meds daily.
- If you limit any normal activity such as walking quickly, climbing stairs, playing hard or singing, you have *severe persistent asthma*. You should see an asthma specialist.

Many people don't know how severe their asthma is. They have become so used to their symptoms that they no longer notice them.

You can tell how severe an **asthma problem** is today by writing the zone of your peak flow or signs score on your asthma diary. A mild problem falls in the High Yellow Zone. A moderate problem falls in the Low Yellow Zone. A severe problem falls in the Red Zone. (see Asthma Diaries on page 28).

If you and your regular doctor cannot get very good control of your asthma, see an asthma specialist.

Peak Flow Meter

The peak flow meter measures the fastest rate at which you can blow air out of your lungs.

If you check your peak flow, you can tell early that you are having a problem. If you treat it right away, you can usually avoid care in the ER.

The peak flow rate often drops before you or your doctor can notice any sign of asthma.

With a peak flow meter, you or your doctor can tell if your air flow has dropped five percent. (Without a peak flow meter, your doctor can't notice any change in airflow until it has dropped 25 percent).

Almost all five-year-olds can learn to use a peak flow meter after they practice at home for a few weeks.

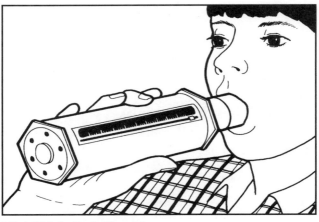

Mini-Wright Peak Flow Meter

How to Use a Peak Flow Meter

You measure your peak flow rate with a peak flow meter. Ask your doctor or nurse to check that you are doing it right:

- Remove gum or food from your mouth.
- Move the pointer to zero.
- Stand up.
- Hold the meter straight.
- Keep your fingers away from the marker and vent holes.
- Open your mouth wide and slowly breathe in as much air as you can.
- Put the mouthpiece flat on your tongue (like a Popsicle) and close your lips tightly around it.
- Blow out as fast as you can — a short, sharp blast.
- Note your score, then move the pointer to zero.
- Wait at least 15 seconds.

Repeat this process two more times. Mark the best score of three on your peak flow diary.

If blowing a peak flow makes you cough, your asthma is not well controlled. Follow your asthma action plan (see page 30).

Getting Peak Flow Right

Blowing peak flow is like competing in the high jump. You count only the best of three tries.

Your score may be falsely high if you:
- spit when you start to blow,
- block the mouthpiece with your tongue before you start to blow or,
- cough when you blow.

This happens most often with meters that have a small mouthpiece. To avoid this problem, put the mouthpiece flat on your tongue. Do not cough when you blow. If you do, you may get a falsely high score even if the mouthpiece is flat on your tongue.

Your score may be falsely low if:
- you blow too slowly,
- you don't hold your lips tightly around the mouthpiece or,
- your fingers block a vent or the marker.

Do not blame low peak flow scores on poor technique or poor effort. If your *technique* is poor on one blow, you should correct it on the next. If your *effort* is poor, you should increase your score on the next blow.

If you can only blow a peak flow in the red zone, you have a serious problem. See a doctor right away.

If you cannot move the marker or it hardly moves, call 911 or go to the ER right away.

Peak Flow Zones

You and your doctor can use peak flow scores to create a plan to treat your asthma. For an example of an Asthma Action Plan based on peak flow, see page 32.

Proper treatment should clear the swelling, narrowing and excess mucus from your airways. Then you can figure out your *personal best* peak flow score. Use this score to define your treatment zones. The zones match the colors of a traffic light.

Green = okay. Scores between 80 and 100 percent of your best score are in the green or okay zone. This means that air moves well through your airways.

If you take a control medicine, you should still take it even if you are in the green zone and feeling fine. This treatment will prevent most signs and symptoms of asthma. It also will make it less likely that you will need care in the ER. The few problems that do happen will be much easier to treat.

High Yellow = caution. Scores between 65 and 79 percent of your personal best are in the high yellow zone. This means you are having a mild problem. Get rid of triggers and change your treatment routine by keeping to your written plan.

Low Yellow = greater caution. Scores between 50 and 64 percent of your personal best are in the low yellow zone and mean you are having a moderate problem. Change your treatment.

Red = danger. If scores are less than 50 percent of your personal best peak flow, take a quick relief med and see your doctor or go to the ER right away.

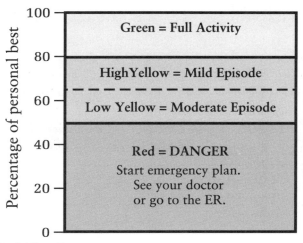

Peak Flow Zones

Asthma Diaries

A well-designed asthma diary can help you learn how triggers and medicines affect your peak flow and asthma symptoms. The asthma peak flow diary will help you to:

- Learn what triggers provoke a problem.
- Track your meds.
- Know when to start and reduce meds.
- See when you are getting better or worse.

This book has a peak flow diary that is more useful than others because:

- The graphic design lets you see peak flow trends at a glance. This helps you take action early.
- There are two yellow zones. Mild asthma problems fall in the high yellow zone. Moderate problems fall in the low yellow zone. A diary with a single yellow zone will not let you know about this change.
- There is space to record signs and symptoms. Sometimes they appear before your peak flow drops.
- The diary lets you see how a change in medicine or triggers affects your peak flow and signs.
- It displays all the facts that your doctor needs to choose the lowest possible dose of inhaled steroids.

- The published diary sheets are in color. This makes it easy to see that you have changed from one zone to another.

A Diary for Children Under Five

Children under five can't blow peak flow well. Instead of peak flow, use the four main signs of asthma to track your child's status. The four signs are cough, wheeze, sucking in the chest skin and breathing faster.

These signs appear early. They change as your child gets better or worse. Since you can hear or see these signs, you can score them. This means you do not have to ask your child. A baby sitter can do the same. To get a total score, add the score for each of the signs. The total score places your child in one of the four asthma treatment zones.

You can find a copy of the Asthma Signs Diary in *Dr. Tom Plaut's Asthma Guide for People of All Ages* or at www.pedipress.com.

Name: **John Mott**

ASTHMA DIARY
PEAK FLOW
For adults, teens & children
five years of age and over

Triggers, Comments

first visit to specialist (above 8/25 column)

O - *Before bronchodilator* X - *After bronchodilator* / Date	8/23	8/24	8/25	8/26	8/27	8/...

Peak Flow Rate

100%	650	
Green Zone	90%	585
	80%	520
High Yellow Zone	70%	455
	65%	420
Low Yellow Zone	60%	390
	50%	325
Red Zone		

Medicines

	8/23	8/24	8/25	8/26	8/27	8/...
med name, dose Inhaled steroid **2 x**	✓✓	✓✓	✓✓	✓✓	✓✓	✓✓
Cromolyn or nedocromil						
med name, dose Adrenaline-like medicine **2-4x**	✓✓ ✓	✓✓ ✓	✓✓ ✓✓	✓✓ ✓	✓✓ ✓	✓✓ ✓
med name, dose Oral steroid **1 x**		✓	✓	✓	✓	✓
med name, dose Theophylline **2 x**	✓✓	✓✓	✓✓	✓✓	✓✓	✓✓

Signs

	8/23	8/24	8/25	8/26	8/27	8/...
Wheeze	1	1	1	0	0	0
Cough	0	0	0	0	0	0
Activity	2	2	2	1	0	1
Sleep	2	2	2	0	0	0

* Fill in the brand name of your medicine, dose, and number of times per da...

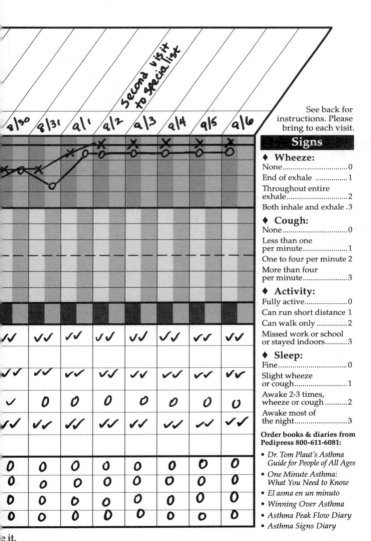

Second visit to specialist

	8/30	8/31	9/1	9/2	9/3	9/4	9/5	9/6
	✓✓	✓✓	✓✓	✓✓	✓✓	✓✓	✓✓	✓✓
	✓✓	✓✓	✓✓	✓✓	✓✓	✓✓	✓✓	✓✓
	✓	0	0	0	0	0	0	0
	✓✓	✓✓	✓✓	✓✓	✓✓	✓✓	✓✓	✓✓
	0	0	0	0	0	0	0	0
	0	0	0	0	0	0	0	0
	0	0	0	0	0	0	0	0
	0	0	0	0	0	0	0	0

See back for instructions. Please bring to each visit.

Signs

♦ **Wheeze:**
None.................................0
End of exhale 1
Throughout entire
exhale...............................2
Both inhale and exhale .3

♦ **Cough:**
None.................................0
Less than one
per minute......................1
One to four per minute 2
More than four
per minute......................3

♦ **Activity:**
Fully active.....................0
Can run short distance 1
Can walk only 2
Missed work or school
or stayed indoors...........3

♦ **Sleep:**
Fine.................................0
Slight wheeze
or cough..........................1
Awake 2-3 times,
wheeze or cough 2
Awake most of
the night..........................3

Order books & diaries from Pedipress 800-611-6081:

e it.
01002 (800) 611-6081. www.pedipress.com

Asthma Action Plans

Ask your doctor to give you a written asthma action plan. It should give the name and dose of each medicine and how often to take it. The four zone asthma action plans on pages 32 and 34 will tell you how to handle every asthma problem:

- When to exercise less.
- When to increase your medicine dose.
- When to add a medicine.
- When to call your doctor.
- When to go to the ER.

The *signs action plan* is used for children under the age of five. Everyone else can use the *peak flow action plan*. This plan is based on your peak flow scores. The four treatment zones are color coded like a traffic light.

You are in the **green zone** and doing well if:

- your peak flow scores are between 80 and 100 percent of your personal best, and
- you have no signs or symptoms and use albuterol less than three days a week.

You may have signs or symptoms when your peak flow is in the green zone. This happens if your zones were set while your airways were inflamed. Increase your treatment to clear your airways. Then reset your zones.

Signs and symptoms may also occur in the green zone when your small airways are inflamed. This does not reduce peak flow. You should start high yellow zone treatment.

You are in the **high yellow zone** and have a mild problem if your peak flow is 65 to 79 percent of your personal best.
- You should avoid triggers and take a quick relief medicine.
- Your plan may also increase the dose of your inhaled steroid.

You are in the **low yellow zone** if your peak flow is between 50 and 64 percent of your personal best.
- If you can't get into the high yellow zone and stay there for four hours after taking albuterol, you are stuck. Call your doctor. You may need to take an oral steroid.

You are in the **red zone** if your peak flow score is less than 50 percent of your personal best.
- If you can't get into the low yellow zone and stay there for four hours after taking albuterol, you are stuck. You need to see your doctor or go to the ER.

A three zone asthma plan has a single yellow zone. It treats someone who is slightly sick the same as someone who is almost ready for care in the ER. When you use a three zone plan, you may miss the chance to prevent an attack from getting worse.

ASTHMA ACTION PLAN – PEAK FLOW

For Adults, Teens and Children Age 5 and Over

Do not guess. Call the doctor if you have any questions about this plan.

Name: _____ Date: _____ Best Peak Flow: _____

Green	**GREEN ZONE: Peak flow score between _____ and _____ .**
	• Fully active.
	• **Med to be taken every day:**
	  ❑ Quick relief medicine _____ (med) : 1 or 2 puffs 15 minutes before exercise.
	
	  ❑ Inhaled steroid _____ : _____ puffs using a holding chamber, **OR** as a dry powder _____ inhaled _____ times a day.
	  ❑ Other _____ : _____ : _____ .
	  ❑ Other _____ : _____ : _____ .

High Yellow	**HIGH YELLOW ZONE: Peak flow score between _____ and _____ , OR if any cough,** wheeze or sign of a cold.
	• Avoid triggers and change meds. No hard exercise.
	• **Meds to be taken:**
	  ❑ Double inhaled steroid dose to: _____ puffs _____ times per day. Take it until your peak flow is in the Green Zone for seven days.
	  ❑ Quick relief med: _____ puffs _____ to _____ times in 24 hours. Take it until your peak flow is in the Green Zone for two days.
	  ❑ Keep taking your other Green Zone meds.

LOW YELLOW ZONE: Peak flow score between _____ and _____.

✓ Take 4 puffs of quick relief med.

✓ **Check your peak flow again in 10 minutes.** If your score has increased into the High Yellow Zone, stay with that plan. Check your peak flow every 1 to 2 hours.

If your score stays in the Low Yellow Zone, or falls back into it in less than 4 hours, **you are stuck.** Follow the Low Yellow Zone plan (below):

☐ Keep treating with High Yellow Zone meds as above.

☐ Add oral steroid _____ mg right away. Take daily until peak flow scores are in the Green Zone for at least 24 hours.

☐ Please call the office before starting oral steroid.

You should improve within two days of treatment and reach the green zone within five days. See your doctor if your progress is slower.

RED ZONE: Peak flow score less than _____.

✓ Take 4 puffs of quick relief med right away.

✓ Take oral steroid _____ mg right away.

✓ Check your peak flow again in 10 minutes.

• If your peak flow score reaches the Low Yellow Zone, follow that plan. Check your peak flow every 1 to 2 hours.

• If your peak flow stays in the Red Zone, or falls back into it within 4 hours, see your doctor or **GO TO THE E.R. RIGHT AWAY.**

Low Yellow

Red

From *Dr. Tom Plaut's Asthma Guide for People of All Ages* by Thomas F. Plaut, MD © Pedipress, Inc. All rights reserved. May be copied for personal or individual use. Written permission required for sale or commercial use. Pedipress, Inc. 125 Red Gate Lane, Amherst, MA 01002.   1.3

33

ASTHMA ACTION PLAN — SIGNS (For Children Under Age 5)

Do not guess. Call the doctor if you have any questions about this plan.

Name: _____

Date: _____

Green

GREEN ZONE: No cough, wheeze, breathing faster or sucking in of the chest skin.

- Fully active.
- Medicine (med) to be taken every day:
  - ☐ Inhaled steroid _____ puffs _____ times a day using a holding chamber with mask.
  - OR
  - _____ ampules _____ times a day by mist machine.
  - ☐ Other _____.

High Yellow

HIGH YELLOW ZONE: Total asthma sign score 1 to 4. Measure this before giving quick relief medicine.

- Avoid triggers. No hard exercise.
- Meds to be taken:
  - ☐ Double inhaled steroid dose. Keep giving until signs score is in the Green Zone for seven days.
  - ☐ Other _____.
  - ☐ Quick relief med: _____.
    - ✓ Give _____ times in 24 hours.* Keep giving until score is _____ for 2 days.

* Start the Low Yellow Zone plan if you need to give quick relief med six times in a day.

Action Plan based on total score of all 4 signs:

Cough:
None 0
Less than 1 per minute 1
1 - 4 per minute 2
More than 4 per minute 3

Wheeze:
None 0
End of exhale 1
Throughout exhale 3
Inhale and exhale 5

Sucking in the chest skin:
None 0
Can hardly see 1
Easy to see 3
Severe 5

Breathing faster:
None 0
A little 1
Some 2
A lot 3

34

LOW YELLOW ZONE: Total asthma sign score 5 to 8.

✓ Give quick relief med _____ puffs using a holding chamber with mask OR one ampule by mist machine.

✓ **Check your child's total signs score again after 10 minutes. If it reaches the High Yellow Zone, follow that plan. Check the signs score every 1 to 2 hours.**

If the score stays in the Low Yellow Zone, or falls back into it in less than 4 hours, add:

☐ Oral steroid _____ mg, _____ cc right away. Give once daily until sign score, when off quick relief med, is _____ for at least 24 hours.

☐ Please call the office before starting oral steroid.

Your child should improve within two days and reach the green zone within five days. See your doctor if your child's progress is slower.

RED ZONE: Total asthma sign score 9 or more.

✓ Give quick relief med _____ puffs using a holding chamber with mask, OR give one ampule by mist machine.

✓ Give oral steroid _____ mg, _____ cc right away.

✓ Check your child's total asthma signs score again in 10 minutes.

If the score reaches the Low Yellow Zone, follow that plan. Check signs scores every 1 to 2 hours.

If your child is still in the Red Zone, or falls back into it in less than 4 hours, visit your doctor OR GO TO THE E.R. RIGHT AWAY.

Low Yellow

Red

Asthma Medicines (meds)

The three major types of asthma meds are called controller (control), quick relief and oral steroid. Take a control med every day if you have signs or symptoms of asthma more than two days a week. Some people need to take more than one control med to control symptoms.

Some control meds block the asthma reaction before it affects the airways. They are:
- Inhaled steroids, leukotriene modifier meds and cromolyn and nedocromil. These meds block the asthma reaction before it affects the airways.

Other control meds can be taken along with inhaled steroids. They reduce the amount of inhaled steroid needed to control asthma symptoms. They are called:
- Long acting $beta_2$-agonist meds. They dilate the airways.

Quick relief meds are used to treat an asthma problem or to prevent symptoms caused by hard exercise. They are also called rescue meds. The quick relief meds are:

- Beta$_2$-agonists. These quickly relax the muscles around the airways.
- Ipratropium. This relaxes the muscles around the airways. It does not act as quickly as a beta$_2$-agonist medicine.

Oral steroids are in a class of their own. They are often used to reduce the swelling in the airways during a moderate or severe asthma problem. They also can be used to treat people with severe persistent asthma whose symptoms can't be controlled any other way.

Each of these meds is described in the pages that follow.

Inhaled Steroids

Med type: Control

Inhaled steroids are the most effective control meds. They prevent asthma problems by blocking inflammation and reducing the sensitivity of the airways. They also reduce swelling in airways that are already inflamed.

These meds include beclomethasone (QVAR), budesonide (Pulmicort), flunisolide (Aerobid), fluticasone (Flovent), mometasone (Asmanex) and triamcinolone (Azmacort).

Possible bad effects:

Minor, *short-term* delay in a child's growth. This does not affect adult height.

Growth of yeast in the mouth.

Hoarseness.

To prevent these effects, use a holding chamber with your inhaler. Also rinse your mouth and spit out after use.

Comments

- The bad effects of taking an inhaled steroid every day for a year are less than those of taking oral steroids every day for two weeks.
- Inhaled steroids may start to work in one day but may take up to four weeks to reach their full effect.
- When you inhale steroids from an inhaler, always use a holding chamber. This will give you the best results.

Long Acting Meds that Dilate the Airways

Med type: Control

These meds help prevent asthma symptoms by keeping the airways open for up to 12 hours.

These meds include:

- Salmeterol (Serevent) comes as a dry powder alone or combined with Flovent (Advair). You inhale these from a blister pack.
- Formoterol (Foradil). You inhale this dry powder med from a capsule.
- Long-acting albuterol (Volmax), a tablet.

Possible bad effects:

Headache, tremor, irregular heartbeat.

Comments

- *Do not use for emergency relief during an asthma episode.*
- Can add to treatment when a standard dose of an inhaled steroid does not control asthma symptoms.
- Can help prevent symptoms through the night.
- Can be taken 30 to 60 minutes before exercise. This will prevent signs and symptoms of asthma for eight to 12 hours.

Leukotriene Modifier Meds

Med type: Control

These meds help prevent asthma symptoms by blocking an early part of the asthma reaction.

They include montelukast (Singulair) and zafirlukast (Accolate).

Possible bad effects:

These include headache, nausea, dizziness, rash, fatigue and stomach ache.

Comments

- Are used to boost the effect of inhaled steroids.
- Sometimes used alone to treat mild persistent asthma.
- Because these meds act slowly, *do not use for emergency relief during an asthma attack.*
- Take tablets once or twice per day (varies with the brand).
- Children's tablet of montelukast can be chewed.
- May be very useful for people who are allergic to aspirin.
- May help to treat allergic rhinitis.

Cromolyn and Nedocromil

Med type: Control

These meds prevent asthma problems by keeping the airways from becoming inflamed. They also keep the muscles around the airways from tightening.

These meds include cromolyn (Intal) and nedocromil (Tilade).

Possible bad effects:

With cromolyn, cough may occur. With nedocromil, you may have a bad taste in your mouth.

Comments

Cromolyn (Intal):

- Produces full effect in one to four weeks.
- Can be used to treat infants.
- Prevents symptoms if taken 5 to 60 minutes before exercise or contact with a dog or cat. Effect lasts three to four hours.

Nedocromil (Tilade):

- Prevents symptoms of chronic asthma in older children and adults. May start to work within 3 days.

For best effect, your doctor may prescribe an oral steroid and rescue med to clear and dilate your airways during the first week of your treatment.

Short Acting Beta$_2$-agonist Meds

Med type: Quick relief

These meds dilate the airways quickly.

They include albuterol (Proventil HFA and Ventolin HFA), levalbuterol (Xopenex), pirbuterol (Maxair) and terbutaline (Bricanyl).

Possible bad effects:

Shakiness or tremor and increased heart rate.

Comments

- These are the fastest, safest and most effective meds used to treat an asthma episode.
- Levalbuterol (Xopenex) is a pure form of albuterol. It lasts longer and causes fewer bad effects than other types of albuterol.

Why should you inhale these meds rather than swallow them?

- Inhaled meds go right into the airways where they act, so you only need a small dose.
- This small dose causes less shakiness.
- They bring relief within a few minutes.
- Meds you swallow often take more than 20 minutes to work. They cause more bad effects because you need to take a much higher dose.

Ipratropium

Med type: Quick relief
This med dilates the airways.
Includes: Ipratropium (Atrovent).
Possible bad effects:
Cough, dry mouth, bad taste.

Comments

- This med acts fast to open the airways. But it is not as fast as a $beta_2$-agonist med.
- Can be inhaled from an inhaler or a mist machine.
- Often added to treatment when a $beta_2$-agonist med does not bring relief of symptoms during an asthma problem.
- Good for people who take a beta-blocker to treat heart disease. They can't use the other quick relief meds.
- If spray or mist hits the eyes, it may make your eyes hurt or make your vision blurry. You can avoid this by using a holding chamber.
- Often used with albuterol (Combivent) to treat chronic obstructive pulmonary disease (COPD).

Oral Steroids

Med type: Unique

These meds open the airways two ways. They reduce the swelling of the inflamed airways. They also decrease the amount of mucus they make.

They help the airways respond better to beta$_2$-agonist meds.

Names of these meds include prednisone, prednisolone and methylprednisolone.

Possible bad effects:

These depend on how much, how often, and how long you take them.

Oral steroids most often are taken for three to seven days, based on asthma signs or peak flow scores. After one day, they may make you hungry, feel good or not able to sleep. People who take oral steroids for more than two weeks may get serious side effects. Talk to your doctor about this.

After you stop taking an oral steroid med, you may be moody for a few days

Comments

- Used to treat moderate or severe problems.
- Rarely needed more than 14 days a year.
- Used for months to treat people with severe persistent asthma if other treatments don't control symptoms.
- These are not the steroids that athletes use to build their muscles.

Antihistamines

A postnasal drip (due to sinus trouble or rhinitis) may trigger asthma symptoms.

Antihistamines dry the nasal passages. They reduce swelling and postnasal drip. When the drip stops, asthma symptoms often decrease.

People with asthma can take these meds safely.

Why does the package warn people with asthma not to use this med?

Doctors used to think that antihistamines would dry the mucus in the airways and make it harder to cough up. This has not been proven.

Cough Meds

If you cough during exercise or at night, your asthma control is poor. Reduce the triggers around you, then follow your asthma action plan. If your cough does not stop, see your doctor.

Do not use a cough medicine instead of your regular asthma medicines.

Taking Inhaled Meds

Inhaled meds go straight into the airways where they work right away. For this reason, you can use them in smaller doses than meds that you swallow. When you use a smaller dose, you will have fewer side effects.

The force, taste and cloud of mist varies from inhaler to inhaler. Some meds have no taste at all.

Prime your inhaler if you haven't used it for a week. Puff it once or twice into the air to make sure you are getting a full puff.

Which Inhaled Med Should You Use First?

If you take more than one med by inhaler, use the quick relief med (that opens the airways) first.

These meds include: albuterol (Proventil HFA and Ventolin HFA), levalbuterol (Xopenex), pirbuterol (Maxair), terbutaline (Bricanyl) and ipratropium (Atrovent).

When you have symptoms, the quick relief med will open the airways wider. Then you can inhale your inhaled steroid deep into your lungs.

How to Use an Inhaler

To get the best effect from your inhaler:
- Hold the mouthpiece one or two inches from your lips.
- Open your mouth wide and breathe out.
- Start to breathe in. *Then* press the little can down.
- Fill your lungs for three to five seconds.
- Hold your breath as long as you can (up to 10 seconds).
- Wait 30 seconds before taking your next puff.
- During a problem, wait one to three minutes between each puff of a quick relief med.

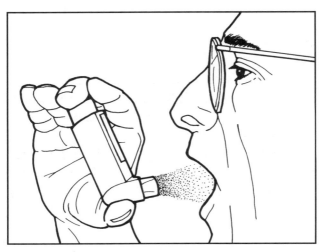

Proper Inhaler Position

Holding Chamber

A holding chamber helps you take meds from an inhaler because:

- It is easy to hold in the right place.
- It holds the puff of med so you can inhale it slowly. This lets more med enter the airway. Less med stays in your mouth.
- It dilutes the bad taste of meds.

Med mist can cause bad effects when it is absorbed from your mouth. Using a holding chamber will reduce this.

Put only one puff of med into the chamber at a time. Wait at least 30 seconds between each puff of med.

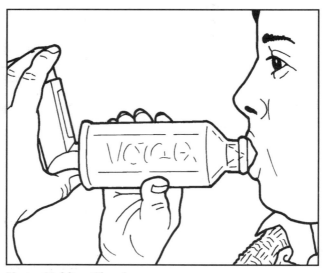

Vortex Holding Chamber

How to Use a Holding Chamber

When you are learning how to use a holding chamber, ask your doctor or nurse to check your technique.

- Shake your inhaler and remove the cap.
- Put the mouthpiece into the holding chamber.
- Breathe out and put the holding chamber mouthpiece flat on your tongue.
- Close your lips tightly around the mouthpiece.
- Spray one puff of med into the chamber.
- Breathe in fully for three to five seconds.
- Hold your breath for 10 seconds.
- Take the chamber out of your mouth and breathe out.
- Wait 30 seconds before you spray a second puff into the chamber.

Comments:
- Do not spray more than one puff at a time into the chamber. If you do, the med droplets will clump and be too large to enter your airways. Because of this, two puffs will help you less than one.
- If your child is having an asthma problem, wait one to three minutes between puffs of a quick relief medicine.

Holding Chamber with Mask

A holding chamber with mask will help any child or adult who cannot hold their breath for ten seconds or has other problems using a holding chamber. When you use a holding chamber with mask, you:

- Get all the benefits of a holding chamber.
- Don't have to hold your breath.
- Can give med to an infant or small child.

It is easy to use even when your child is quite sick.

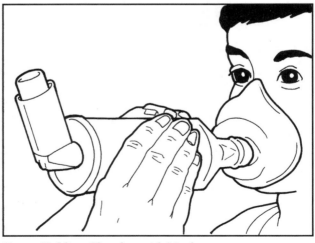

Vortex Holding Chamber with Mask

How to Use a Holding Chamber with Mask

When you are learning to use a holding chamber with mask, ask your doctor or nurse to check your technique.

- Shake the inhaler and remove the cap.
- Put the inhaler mouthpiece into the end of the holding chamber.
- Place the mask tightly over your child's nose and mouth. It must make a good seal with the skin.
- Spray one puff of med into the holding chamber.
- Let your child breathe in and out for six normal breaths. An adult should breathe in and out for three normal breaths.
- Wait 30 seconds before you spray a second puff into the chamber.

Comments

- Masks come in several sizes.
- If your child is having an asthma problem, wait one to three minutes between puffs of a quick relief medicine.
- Do not spray more than one puff at a time into the chamber. If you do, the med droplets will clump and be too large to enter the airways. Taking two puffs at once will help you less than taking one puff at a time.

Breath Actuated Inhaler

Many people like these inhalers better than the others. Your breath triggers the release of med from this device.

- Raise the lever until it snaps into place.
- Shake the inhaler and breathe out.
- Close your lips tightly around the mouthpiece.
- Inhale deeply with a steady, medium force.
- After you hear a click, keep breathing in for three to five seconds.
- Hold your breath for ten seconds, then breathe out slowly.
- Lower the lever after each puff.

Do not use this inhaler with a holding chamber.

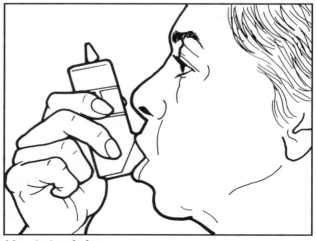

Maxair Autohaler

Is Your Inhaler Empty?

You can figure out how many days your new inhaler will last. To do this, first find the total number of puffs in the little can (this is written on the label). Then, divide that number by the number of puffs you take each day. For example, if the can has 120 puffs and you take two puffs a day, it will last 60 days. Write the discard date on the can.

Other ways of checking if your inhaler has enough med are not helpful. The shake test doesn't work, the puff test wastes medicine and the float test plugs the valve stem of some inhalers and makes them useless.

Dry Powder Inhaler

You can inhale some asthma meds as a dry powder. The powder is stored in foil blisters, capsules or in the body of the inhaler. You suck the powder into your lungs when you breathe in. Many people find a dry powder inhaler easier to use than a mist inhaler.

Some benefits of using a dry powder are:
• There is no problem with position or timing.
• A counter tells when it is empty.
• They do not damage the ozone layer as some mist inhalers do.

How to Use the Turbuhaler Dry Powder Inhaler (DPI)

- Hold the Turbuhaler with the mouthpiece facing up. Turn the brown grip to the right as far as it will go. Then twist the grip to the left until it clicks.
- Turn your head away and breathe out.
- Close your lips tightly around the mouthpiece.
- Take a deep, fast breath in through your mouth. (You do not need to hold your breath.)
- Remove the Turbuhaler from your mouth.
- If your doctor has prescribed more than one dose, wait 30 seconds and repeat.
- Rinse your mouth and spit out after use.

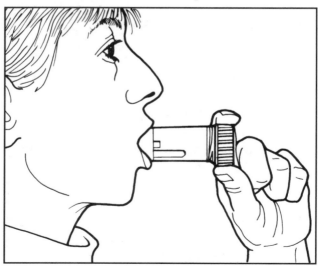

Using a Turbuhaler Dry Powder Inhaler

How to Use the Diskus (DPI)

- Hold the Diskus dry powder inhaler flat. The label should be facing up.
- Expose the mouthpiece and a small lever.
- Press the small lever over to the dose counter until you hear it click.
- Turn your head away and breathe out.
- Close your lips tightly around the mouthpiece.
- Breathe in steadily and deeply through your mouth.
- Remove the Diskus from your mouth.
- Hold your breath for 10 seconds.
- Close the Diskus by rotating the thumb grip.
- Rinse your mouth and spit out after use.

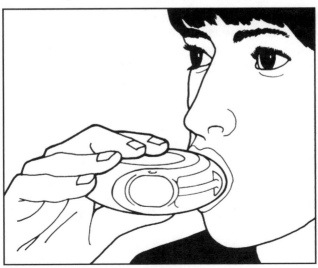

Using a Diskus Dry Powder Inhaler

Compressor Driven Nebulizer (Mist Machine)

A mist machine changes liquid meds into a cloud of mist.

Use your mist machine if you find it easier than using an inhaler with holding chamber.

Treatment should take 4 to 12 minutes. This varies with the cup and machine that you use.

- For best results use a mouthpiece.
- Place the mouthpiece flat on your tongue (like a Popsicle)
- Close your lips tightly around it.
- A mask may help some very young children and "nose breathers." Be sure the mask rests tightly on your child's face.
- Don't hold the mouthpiece or mask away from the face. This "blow by" technique delivers only a very small amount of med to the lungs.

After you inhale the med mist, it must settle in your airways. To help this happen:

- Breathe slowly, (10 to 20 times a minute) if possible.
- Breathe in slower than you breathe out.

Nebulizer cups vary greatly in quality. A really good cup can deliver three times as much med as most of the cups that are sold.

For best results, buy a cup that:
- Makes most of the mist the right size to enter the airways (1 to 5 microns).
- Loses very little mist on exhale.

The reusable cups made by Pari Respiratory can do this. Be sure to replace them every six months.

Ultrasonic nebulizers are used the same way as compressor driven nebulizers. They weigh less, run more quietly and cost much more. However, they destroy inhaled steroids and should not be used to deliver them.

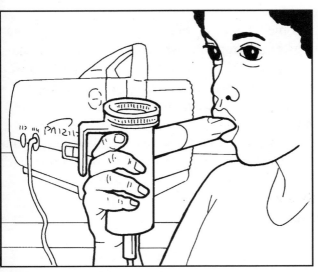

Pari LC Plus Nebulizer Cup

Meds that May Make Asthma Worse

Aspirin and other drugs used to treat **arthritis** may cause asthma symptoms. Some brands are Motrin, Advil, Naprosyn, Daypro and Indocin. About ten percent of adults with asthma have symptoms after they take these meds.

If you take a beta-blocker for **high blood pressure, angina** or **migraine headaches**, it may make your asthma worse. For example, if you start taking a beta-blocker, you may start to cough or wheeze. This can happen even if you never had asthma symptoms before. Some brands of beta-blockers are Lopressor, Corgard, Inderal and Tenormin.

People who have **glaucoma** may find they have worse asthma symptoms when they start to use beta-blocker eye drops. If you use just one drop of this medicine daily, you may get a cough or wheeze. Some brands of these eye drops are Betoptic and Timoptic.

If these meds make your asthma worse, ask your doctor to prescribe a type of med that does not cause asthma symptoms.

You Can Control Your Asthma

More than 2,000,000 people have learned to manage their asthma at home. They know how asthma works in their bodies and how to use the meds and tools their doctors prescribe. You can learn to.

- You can work out an effective asthma action plan with your doctor, nurse or respiratory therapist.
- Using this plan as a guide, you will be able to lead a fully active life.

About the Author

Thomas F. Plaut, M.D. has cared for thousands of people with asthma. He is a nationally known asthma specialist and the author of several books for patients, parents and professionals.

He has developed a distance learning program for allied health professionals, the *One Minute Asthma Training*. It has been used to train school nurses, office nurses and asthma case managers nationwide. (See www.pedipress.com).

Dr. Plaut consults with patients, parents, HMOs, physicians and health organizations. He is on the editorial board of *Advance for Managers of Respiratory Care*.

He sees patients at his office in Amherst, Massachusetts.

Asthma Stories

The Light Bulb

Do you call an electrician when a light bulb burns out?

No. You can change the bulb yourself.

Do you call a doctor when you have an asthma episode?

- If you have worked out a written action plan with your doctor, you can take care of most asthma problems at home.

The Runner

One of my twelve-year-old patients runs the half mile. Her coach thought she was very good.

What happened after she started to use her albuterol (quick relief) inhaler before running? Her times dropped and the coach realized she was excellent.

- Pretreatment may allow you to compete at a higher level.

Fighting Asthma

Suppose your house is on fire.

Do you want the fire fighters to squirt a little water on it and then wait to see if the fire goes out? No.

Suppose you have an asthma attack.

Do you want to use a little medicine and wait to see if the attack stops?

- Intensive treatment will control an attack more safely and quickly.

The Umbrella

When it rains, an umbrella can keep you dry.

Do you close it while it is still raining? No. You will get wet.

Asthma "control" medicines work like an umbrella. They protect you from symptoms and episodes.

- Symptoms often return if you stop the control medicine.

Resource Section

Pedipress Books, Diaries and Management Tools

Pedipress, Inc.
125 Red Gate Lane
Amherst, MA 01002
Toll free: (800) 611-6081
Tel: (413) 549-7798
Fax: (413) 549-4095
www.pedipress.com

Dr. Tom Plaut's Asthma Guide for People of All Ages
Thomas F. Plaut, M.D.
with Teresa B. Jones, M.A.
1999, 310 pages with 120 illustrations, tables and forms. $15.00.

Comprehensive, accurate, and current guide for people who want to understand and control their asthma. Includes complete discussion of the basics of asthma and the medicines used to treat it.

Provides detailed descriptions of inhalation devices, peak flow monitoring, and the use of asthma diaries and asthma action plans. Includes first-person stories by patients who gained control over their asthma. Addresses asthma issues faced in the school, the family and in travel. Includes a resource section, glossary and index.

One Minute Asthma
Thomas F. Plaut, M.D.
2005. 64 pages, $5.00.

Accurate, clear and easy to read. Covers the basics of asthma and the medicines used to treat it. An ideal book for patients, parents, teachers, coaches, friends, relatives and baby-sitters starting to learn about asthma.

El asma en un minuto
Thomas F. Plaut, M.D.
2001. 60 pages, $5.00.
Spanish version of *One Minute Asthma*.

Winning Over Asthma
Eileen Dolan Savage
2001. 40 pages, $7.00.

This picture book presents asthma facts while telling the story of five-year-old Graham.

Asthma Peak Flow Diary
Thomas F. Plaut, M.D.
Three colors, pad of 25 sheets, $5.00.

An ideal learning and monitoring tool for patient and parents who want to understand and control asthma. Also available in Spanish.

Asthma Signs Diary
Thomas F. Plaut, M.D.
Three colors, pad of 25
sheets, $5.00.
Learning and monitoring
tool for children under
five years of age.

Asthma Charts & Forms
for the Physician's Office
and Managed Care
Thomas F. Plaut, M.D. and
Teresa B. Jones, M.A.
76 pages, 2003, $95.00.
Forms save time and
improve patient
compliance. Includes CD
for customizing forms.

One Minute Asthma
Training
Thomas F. Plaut, M.D.
2003. A distance learning
program for allied health
professionals. $995.00 for
a group of six, includes
books and devices.

Healthy Schools
Network

777 Madison Avenue
Albany, NY 12208
(518) 462-0632
www.healthyschools.org
The Healthy Schools
Network is a national
organization centered on
children's environmental
health and dedicated to
assuring every child and
school employee an
environmentally safe and
healthy school.

National Asthma
Education and
Prevention
Program

NHLBI Information
Center
PO Box 30105
Bethesda, MD 20824-0105
(301) 592-8573
www.nhlbi.nih.gov
The NAEPP publishes
information for health
professionals, schools
and the public. Order the
Practical Guide for the
Diagnosis and
Management of Asthma
and other resources by
phone, or download from
the web:
www.nhlbi.nih.gov/
nhlbi/lung/asthma/prof/
practgde.htm

U.S. Environmental
Protection Agency

Indoor Air Quality
Information
Clearinghouse
P.O. Box 37133
Washington, DC 20013-
7133
(800) 438-4318
www.epa.gov/iaq
Publishes information on
indoor air quality in the
home, the school and the
workplace. This includes,
Indoor Air Quality: Tools
for Schools.

Order Form

	Qty	Cost
Dr. Tom Plaut's Asthma Guide for People of All Ages 1999. 310 pages. $15. 6 copies, $10 each.	_____	_____
One Minute Asthma: What You Need to Know 2005. 64 pages. $5. 100 copies, $0.99 each.	_____	_____
El asma en un minuto 2001. Spanish version of *One Minute Asthma*. Similar contents. 60 pages. $5. 100 copies, $0.99 each.	_____	_____
Winning Over Asthma Third edition, 2001. 34 pages. $7.	_____	_____
Asthma Peak Flow Diary 3 colors, 25 sheets per pad. $5. Please specify English or Spanish.	_____	_____
Asthma Signs Diary 3 colors, 25 sheets per pad. $5.	_____	_____

For shipping costs outside the U.S., email info@pedipress.com, **fax** (413) 549-4095 or **call** (800) 611-6081.

Visit www.pedipress.com for discount prices on 100 or more copies.

Subtotal: _____

5% Sales Tax: _____
(Mass. Only)

10% Shipping: _____
($5 min. charge)

Total Enclosed: _____

Name _____

Street _____

City _____ State _____ Zip _____

Telephone _____

Email _____

❏ Mastercard ❏ Visa # _____

Exp. Date _____ Signature _____

Send check, money order or credit card information to:

Pedipress Asthma Publications
125 Red Gate Lane
Amherst, MA 01002
Phone: 800-611-6081; Fax: 413-549-4095
www.pedipress.com